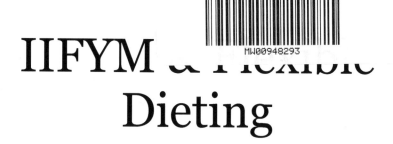

IIFYM & Flexible Dieting

The Easy Way to Burn Fat & Build Muscle Eating the Foods You Love

Colt Milton
(206) 743-1346

Thomas Rohmer

Disclaimer:

This guide has been created for informational and reference
purposes only. The author, publisher, and any other
affiliated parties cannot be held in any way accountable for
any personal injuries or damage allegedly resulting from the
information contained herein, or from any misuse of such
guidance. Although strict measures have been taken to
provide accurate information, the parties involved with the
creation and publication of this guide take no responsibility
for any issues that many arise from alleged discrepancies
contained herein. It is strongly recommended that you
consult a physician, personal trainer, and nutritionist prior
to commencing this or any other workout or diet plan. This
guide is not a substitute for professional personal guidance
from a qualified medical professional. If you feel pain or
discomfort at any point during exercises contained herein,
cease the activity immediately and seek medical guidance.

Table of Contents

Introduction:

It doesn't matter what your fitness goal is. Nutrition can get boring quickly regardless of whether you're trying to burn fat or build muscle. You're tired of gimmicky diets that leave you starving all day. And you're tired of eating chicken breast and broccoli all of the time. Not too long ago, this was the only way people knew how to get in shape. Luckily, there's a much better option available to you and that's if it fits your macros (IIFYM), aka flexible dieting. IIFYM gives you the best of both worlds:

-It's guaranteed to help you reach your goals when properly set up (more on this later).

-And it allows you to do so while eating your favorite foods.

The idea of losing weight by eating ice cream might seem like a crazy idea to you right now and that's ok. By the end of this book, you'll understand the simple science behind how your body works in regards to burning fat and building muscle. You'll also learn what a macronutrient is and the importance of each macronutrient. Finally, you'll have all the tools you need to set up your own flexible diet, track your macros, and get great results from it.

Side note: You'll see me use the terms IIFYM and flexible dieting throughout this book. These are two different words to describe the same thing, and they are interchangeable.

Chapter 1: What the Heck is a Macro Anyway?

What is a Macro Anyway?

Macro is short for macronutrient, and they're basically nutrients that provide the body with energy. The body then uses this energy to carry out all of its processes such as: breathing, organ function, digestion, moving, and a whole lot more. There are three macronutrients: protein, carbohydrates, and fat. Of the three, people consider protein to be superior, fat should be eaten in moderation, and carbs are downright evil.

However, the reality is that this isn't true at all. Each macro has its own importance or else it wouldn't exist. And while you can certainly argue that one is better than the other, at the end of the day, you still need all three to be successful at losing weight or building muscle. Not to be confused with macronutrients, there is also something called micronutrients.

Micronutrients are nutrients needed in trace amounts for normal growth and development in living organisms. They include things such as vitamins and minerals. For the scope of this book, our focus will be on macronutrients. Let's go ahead and break down the importance of each one individually.

Protein

First of all, I think that it's very important to define exactly what protein is. Protein is the most popular of the three macronutrients, and one gram of protein contains 4 calories. Protein is the body's building block for things such as hair, skin, bones, and of course muscle. Protein has many more functions than the ones listed here, but for the purpose of this book I want to focus on protein and its relation to muscle.

Protein is made up of amino acids, which come together in different patterns to form specific proteins with different characteristics. Of the 20 amino acids, 9 are essential, which means that they aren't produced by the body and must be consumed through the diet. A complete protein is a protein that contains all 9 of the essential amino acids in an adequate amount. Some examples of complete proteins are: fish, eggs, milk, and meat.

However, don't worry about if the protein source you're eating is complete or incomplete. Most of the time you'll be consuming an incomplete protein with something else that will cover the missing amino acid(s).

Common Myths About Protein

There are definitely a lot of misconceptions that surround protein these days. No doubt with a lot of mass media attention, there's bound to be some misunderstandings. Not to worry though, the truth will be revealed shortly.

Myth #1: You must eat protein every couple of hours to maintain muscle mass.

One common belief is that you must consume protein every 2-3 hours to prevent your body from becoming catabolic and breaking down muscle mass. This, however, did not turn out to be true in a study done by the American Journal of Clinical Nutrition (1). The study was conducted by taking a group of healthy men and women and then having them consume all of their daily calories in either 1 or 3 meals for a total of 8 weeks.

Guess what the researchers found? They found that there was no difference in the lean body mass of the test subjects. This means that it doesn't matter if you consume all of your protein in one meal. As long as you consume enough protein to meet your daily requirements, you won't lose muscle mass. Hopefully this comes as a relief to you because it would be really annoying if you had to consume protein every couple of hours just to maintain your muscle! It would also defeat the purpose of IIFYM because you'd be forced to stop whatever you're doing and eat protein. How inconvenient!

Myth #2 You Must Consume Protein Immediately After Your Workout to Build Muscle

This is another very common misconception in the fitness industry, and it makes sense as to why. If you want more muscle, then you consume protein soon after your workout because that workout just stimulated the growth of some muscle. However, is it possible to build muscle if you don't immediately consume post workout protein? The answer to that is yes.

Would it make sense if your body pretended like you never worked out in the first place all because you waited a couple of hours before you consumed any protein? This doesn't seem logical, but if you don't believe me, here's another study to back up my claims.

General Nutrition Centers (GNC) conducted a study where people would perform weight-training exercises for 12 weeks (2). The test subjects would then immediately consume 1 of 4 different supplements following the weight workout. The supplements were: protein, creatine with colostrum, protein with creatine, and protein with colostrum.

The groups taking post workout protein gained 2 pounds of muscle in that 12-week period, while the groups consuming creatine post workout gained roughly 5 pounds. This 2-5 pound increase is still typical (not better) of how much you can expect to gain in a 2-4 month period of lifting weights on a solid program without extra supplements (3).

This isn't to say that you should never consume post workout protein; I want you to realize it is ok if you miss it sometimes. Consider your goals and act accordingly. For example, if your goal is to build muscle, then consume post workout protein. However, if you want to burn fat, then you can certainly get by without it.

Too many times people will workout, burn a fair amount of calories, and then they'll completely wipe it away by drinking a post workout shake. If weight loss is the goal, then you need to consume less calories not more (I'll explain this point in more detail later)!

Myth #3 Your Body Can Only Digest 30 Grams of Protein per Meal

It's a good thing that this isn't true, or else you really would have to consume protein every couple of hours just so your body could digest it! Your body will digest, absorb, and utilize all of the protein that you consume in one meal. Your body will first use the protein to replenish amino acid pools, and then if there is excess, that protein will get converted into glycogen.

This glycogen will then get stored in the muscle cells or liver. Also, remember the earlier study where the test subjects consumed all of their daily protein needs in one meal. Their bodies utilized all of the protein from that one meal, not just 30 grams of it.

Is Protein More Important Than Carbs or Fat?

The answer to the above question can really be yes or no. It depends on what you're referring to by 'more important.' All three of the macronutrients are essential, and each macronutrient has a specific function in the body. Fat, for example, is an insulator for the body and stores energy for later use.

Carbs are the body's first source of energy, help with the production of serotonin, and are necessary for the muscles (including the heart), brain, kidneys, and central nervous system to function properly. When you think of the question from this angle, the answer really is no because all 3 macronutrients are important for one reason or another. Nevertheless, let me offer you another perspective to view the question from. Which macronutrient is most important in terms of building muscle?

In this instance, I would have to give the edge to protein. Protein is the building block for body tissue (including muscle), and it can even be used as a source of energy when carb and fat stores are low. Without it, you and your muscles would not exist. Of course, keep in mind that consuming only protein isn't ideal for building muscle. You also need to be consuming carbohydrates and fat to help optimize the muscle building process.

Carbohydrates

As of late, carbs have been getting severely bashed for causing weight gain. There are many myths surrounding carbs making them appear to be more evil than the devil. However, all of this hate is certainly not justified. Let's bust some common myths surrounding carbs.

Common Misconceptions About Carbohydrates

It's very easy to get confused about carbs simply because of all of the myths and flat out lies that are being talked about in the fitness community. Not to fear, many of the stories that you've probably heard aren't true. So let's go ahead and set the record straight.

Myth #1: If You Eat Any Carbs at Night, They'll Automatically Get Stored as Fat

The main premise behind this myth is that your metabolism begins to slow down later in the day when you're getting ready for bed. If you eat carbs late at night, then your metabolism won't have the chance to burn them off like it normally would if you ate that meal earlier in the day. In theory, this makes sense, but it isn't true.

If you're burning off more calories than you consume (i.e. caloric deficit), it doesn't matter if you eat carbs before going to bed. Those late night carbs won't get stored as fat. In fact, it's possible to store carbs as fat even if you ate them during the daytime. This can happen when you're consuming more calories than you're burning off (i.e. caloric surplus). The caloric deficit and surplus are critical concepts you must understand to be successful with fitness. I briefly mentioned them here to illustrate a point, but a much more through explanation will be provided in the next chapter.

Myth #2: Carbs that Rank High on the Glycemic Index Scale are Bad

If you don't know what the glycemic index scale is, it basically measures a food's effect on blood-sugar levels. The higher a food item is on the scale, the faster it will cause a rise in your blood-sugar levels. When your blood sugar levels are high, your body must release a lot of insulin to help shuttle the glucose eaten in the meal to your cells. When your insulin levels are high, your body will be burning off sugar for fuel instead of fat.

Once again, if you're in a caloric deficit, then it doesn't matter if you eat foods that are high on the glycemic index. This is because you're burning off more calories than you're consuming, which means that your body is going to have to use fat (i.e. stored energy) for fuel.

Myth #3: Fruit is Bad for You

This one seems really absurd to me. You hear all of the time about how you should eat more fruits and vegetables, but some people still believe that fruit can be bad for you. This is because fruit contains the simple sugar fructose, and this sugar can be harmful to you when consumed in large quantities. However, most people are never going to consume enough fruit to where this will become a problem. Also, if you're in a caloric deficit, then it doesn't really matter how much fruit you consume. Are you starting to notice a pattern here?

Benefits and Functions of Carbs

Now that I have dispelled some of the common myths about carbohydrates, I'm going to discuss some of the essential benefits that carbs can provide for you. Of the three macronutrients, carbs are your body's first source of energy. When you exercise, your body will burn off carbs and use them to help give your body the necessary energy it needs to complete your workout. Without carbohydrates, your body will start to run low on energy and you'll become more irritable.

If you've ever tried a low carb diet for any significant period of time, you've probably started to notice both of these things occurring. That's the main reason why I don't feel that the low carb diet is a very good long-term weight loss solution.

Not to mention that it's going to be very hard to go the rest of your life without eating any of your favorite carbohydrate rich foods! Another huge benefit of eating plenty of complex carbohydrates is that they are generally high in fiber.

Fiber is important for your digestive health, and it can prevent or relieve you from constipation. Fiber can also lower the risk for developing diabetes and heart disease. So if you need more fiber in your diet, look no further than carbohydrates!

Are Carbs the Real Evil at Hand?

The answer to the above question is probably not. What is at fault for weight gain is overeating of food in general because it's so convenient and easy to do. Since you're reading this, you probably don't think much about how you're going to get your next meal. If you get hungry, you simply prepare your meal or drive somewhere to buy it. With food at your fingertips 24/7, it becomes super easy to eat more than is necessary.

In the hunter and gather days, you had to earn your meal by killing something or at the very least walking somewhere. That's definitely not the case in today's world. If you get hungry, the nearest fast food restaurant is more than likely less than 10 minutes away. Not only that, but the food that you'll be eating at this fast food restaurant will be fairly high in calories. This overabundance and overconsumption of food is the real problem for people gaining weight, not carbs.

Fat

As with carbs, fat has gotten a bad rep over the years. Low fat diets were very popular in the 1990's and early 2000's. Now days, fat is overshadowed for being labeled "the worst macronutrient" in place of carbs. Let's take a closer look at this macronutrient and see if fat truly makes people fat.

We are Hardwired to Like Fat

Did you know that there's actually a reason why you enjoy eating salty and sugary foods that contain a high amount of fat in them? It's simply because this is how we were made! Think back to our ancestors in the hunter and gather days. Back then, calories were scarce and hard to come by. When our ancestors had a chance to eat, it needed to be a big meal high in calories because nobody knew when the next meal might come.

Therefore, our ancestors were drawn to salty and sugary foods that contained lots of fat because these food items were higher in calories than blueberries that could be picked from a bush. Being hardwired to enjoy fatty foods has allowed us to survive for this long, so don't think of it as a bad thing. Of course, in the present day, we typically don't have to worry about running out of food and starving. In fact, we're constantly surrounded and bombarded by food. Needless to say, people back in the day didn't have it so easy.

Functions of Fat

Believe it or not, fat has many different *necessary* functions in the body. You must have at least some stored fat in order to survive. If your body didn't have any stored fat, you would be in trouble as soon as your carb stores get depleted! One of fat's main jobs is to act as an insulator to help maintain a normal body temperature. Fat can also be used as a source of energy when carbohydrate stores are depleted, and fat plays a role in your body's testosterone levels. So don't go on a low fat diet if you want to optimize your testosterone levels!

Common Myths About Fat

Now let's dive into some of the common misunderstandings about fat. These are some of the reasons why many people are afraid to consume an adequate amount of fat on a regular basis. However, fat is your friend, not your enemy. Hopefully after exposing these myths, you'll have a better understanding as to why this is.

Myth #1 Eating Fat Makes You Fat

I can understand why this makes sense to some people. If you eat a diet that's high in fat, then surely that would make you fat right? Wrong. As long as you're in a caloric deficit (i.e. burning off more calories than your consuming), you won't gain weight no matter how many grams of fat you're consuming. So focus on creating a caloric deficit instead of worrying about how much fat you're consuming.

Myth #2 All Types of Fat Are Bad for You

This couldn't be further from the truth. Unsaturated (including mono and polyunsaturated) and even saturated fats are good for you and should be part of your diet. Some research suggests that trans fat is bad for your health (4), but if consumed in moderation, it really can't do much harm. My suggestion would be to not get caught up in what type of fat you're eating all of the time, but to instead focus on the total amount of calories you're consuming.

Myth #3 Fat is Bad for Your Cholesterol

Yes it's bad to have high cholesterol, specifically high LDL (low density lipoprotein) levels. However, if you look at most people who have high cholesterol levels, they usually share one thing in common. What is that, you say? Well it's that they are generally overweight or obese.

People who maintain a healthy bodyweight for their height normally have healthy cholesterol levels. So instead of blaming fat for making you have high cholesterol levels, blame it on an overindulgence in calories.

Is Fat to Blame for the Obesity Epidemic?

With 2/3's of Americans either being overweight or obese, it's easy to blame fat for causing the problem. I mean one gram of fat contains 9 calories compared to only 4 calories per gram for protein and carbs. So it's easier to overeat calories from fat than the other 2 macronutrients. However, fat itself really isn't the problem. What is the main problem? Well it's overeating calories in general from all 3 macronutrients, not just fat itself. As I mentioned earlier, the world we live in today makes it very easy to get food basically whenever we want. When you go on your lunch break from work, you can drive in your car to any convenient fast food restaurant, and I'm willing to bet that whatever you get at that restaurant isn't going to be low in calories. This is much different from the way our ancient ancestors lived. Fast forward back to today, and it's a double whammy. Not only do we not have to exercise to in a sense "earn" our food, but most of the foods we eat are really high in calories. So needless to say, fat actually isn't the issue here.

You should now have a good understanding of each of the three macronutrients. You probably noticed me talking a lot about the caloric deficit; yes, it really is that important! Before we can get into your IIFYM diet, you must first understand how your body burns fat and builds muscle. Most people don't know about this, and they fail because of it. They will blindly eat healthy foods and hope for the best. As you can probably guess, that doesn't work out so well.

Chapter 2: Know Your End Game With IIFYM

Before you can set up a successful flexible diet, you must first know what it is you want to achieve. Do you want to burn fat, lean down, and/or get ripped abs? If so, then your IIFYM diet will look much different from someone who wants to build lean muscle mass. The basics of weight loss and building muscle involve calories. You must first understand what calories are and how they work with your body.

What the Heck is a Calorie Anyway?

Here is the literal definition of a calorie:

"The amount of heat required at a pressure of one atmosphere to raise the temperature of one gram of water one degree Celsius that is equal to about 4.19 joules"

Wow! That sure is a mouthful. Essentially, a calorie is just energy. When you eat calories, you're giving your body energy. This energy is used to fuel all of the chemical reactions (i.e. your metabolism) that occur in your body to sustain life. It takes energy for your body to digest food, maintain organ function, breathe, keep warm, and a lot of other things.

You don't just use energy (i.e. burn calories) by exercising. In fact, the majority of calories you'll burn in a given day will come from your resting metabolic rate (RMR) and not from exercise. Your RMR is the amount of calories that you burn in a day while at rest. Here's a simple formula you can use to determine your RMR:

Bodyweight (in pounds) x13=RMR

Let's use myself as an example:

Weight=200 pounds

200 x13= 2,600 calories

This number is cool and all, but how does it pertain to you losing or gaining weight?

This is How You Gain/Lose Weight

The principle of weight loss/gain is very simple. It's a matter of the 1st law of thermodynamics or energy in vs. energy out:

"If you burn off more calories than you consume, you'll lose weight (i.e. caloric deficit)."

"If you burn off less calories than you consume, you'll gain weight (i.e. caloric surplus)."

Your RMR is very important because it will be the basis for determining how much you need to eat to reach your goal.

In my case with a RMR of 2,600 calories:

- If I eat less than 2,600 calories, I'll lose weight.
- If I eat more than 2,600 calories, I'll gain weight.
- If I eat right at 2,600 calories, I'll maintain my weight.

Weight loss doesn't need to get any more complicated than this.

Side Note: There are approximately 3,500 calories in one pound of fat (5). Meaning that you must create a caloric deficit of 3,500 calories to lose one pound. You can divide 3,500 by 7 days in a week to get 500. Thus if you eat at a caloric deficit of 500 calories daily, you'll lose one pound per week. Using my example again:

RMR=2,600
2,600-500=2,100

So if I eat 2,100 calories on a daily basis, I'll start losing 1 pound per week.

What should you do to burn off more calories than you consume and create a caloric deficit? The answer to that is simple as well; eat less and/or move more. I say and/or because you don't have to exercise to lose weight. You could also exercise more and lose weight without any change to your diet.

However, for most people, exercising more simply won't be enough. Diet is the easiest (and fastest) way to manipulate your total calories. But what diet is the best? Obviously I have a bias towards flexible dieting, but as you're about to find out, all diets try to achieve the same goal. Some fail at this miserably (low carb, liquid diet, etc.), while others can leave you with lasting success (flexible dieting, of course).

All Diets Try to Achieve This

As you learned earlier, the only way that you can lose weight is by creating a caloric deficit. Believe it or not, this is actually the goal of every diet that's ever existed. This agenda is disguised in different forms depending on what the diet is.

For example, with the low carb diet, you're reducing the total amount of calories you're eating by consuming less carbs. If you're on a diet where you eat nothing but "healthy foods," then you're reducing your calories by eliminating things that are higher in calories for foods lower in calories. Yet there are three main reasons why diets like this are terrible:

1. They make you miserable- giving up carbs and eliminating your favorite foods isn't fun
2. They don't guarantee weight loss- you can still overeat healthy foods
3. They're not sustainable- are you really going to go the rest of your life without ice cream, burgers, or whatever else it is that you like?

In the end, there isn't a best diet that will work for everyone. You have to follow one rule: burn off more calories than you consume. Whatever diet plan makes it the easiest for you to follow that rule for an extended period of time is the best diet for you. Fortunately, IIFYM is very easy to do and maintain for life. People have lost weight trying everything under the sun, but the key is whether or not they able to keep the weight off. Most of the time the answer is no.

What if Your Goal is to Build Muscle?

If your doing IIFYM to build muscle, then your diet strategy is going to look different from someone who's looking to lose weight. The main difference will come down to the amount of calories you'll eat. While the person who wants to lose weight will be creating a caloric deficit, you'll be in a caloric surplus.

You must eat more than you burn off and give your body the raw materials it needs in order to build muscle. Think of it this way. Let's say you go on a 200-mile road trip. In order to drive the 200 miles, you'll need a certain amount of gas. Without the proper amount of gas, you'll run out of fuel and have to stop your trip short of where you want to go.

The same is true with building muscle. You need a certain amount of fuel, calories, in order to give your body enough of the building blocks it needs to add more muscle mass.

The trick with building muscle is to not go overboard with the calories. Eating too much will lead to excess fat gain. Up to a certain point with weight loss, you can eat less and less and lose weight at that much faster of a pace. The same isn't true for building muscle. Eating more and more calories will not lead to more muscle gains. You're body will use what it needs, and then it will store the rest as fat.

The question then becomes, how big of a caloric surplus should you eat? The sad reality is that the muscle building process is very slow. As a natural, you can expect to gain about .5 pound of muscle per week (6). That may not seem like a lot, but if you strategically build muscle in the right places (upper chest, shoulders, and back), this will add up quickly and have a profound effect on your physique. The trick is being consistent. If you multiply .5 by 52 weeks in a year, you'll add 26 pounds of muscle to your frame. That will make a huge difference to your physique!

In order to gain half a pound per week, you'll need to add 250 to your RMR. This will put you in a caloric surplus, and it'll give your body the necessary nutrients to pack on muscle. Using the example from above:

RMR=2,600 calories
2,600+250= 2,850 calories

This means I'll need to eat roughly 2,850 calories on a daily basis in order to gain half a pound of muscle per week.

Chapter 3: The Basics of IIFYM

Now it's time for the fun part. We're going to set up your IIFYM diet. Essentially, we're going to figure out exactly how many grams of carbs, protein, and fat you need to be eating on a daily basis. From there, you'll simply eat that much and start seeing results. It really is that simple.

The cool part is that you're technically allowed to eat whatever you want as long as it fits within your macro parameters (more on this point later). For example, let's say you determined you needed to eat 150 grams of carbs, 150 grams of protein, and 50 grams of fat everyday to start losing weight. You can mix and match and eat any combination of foods you like as long as it fits within your macros. This means that if you eat French toast and it contains 100 grams of carbs you only have 50 grams of carbs you're allowed to eat for the rest of the day. If you go above 50, you're breaking the only rule of flexible dieting—don't overeat a macronutrient.

Before we can get into how much of each macro you need to eat, it's critical you know the following information:

1. What is your resting metabolic rate (RMR)? You can find your RMR by multiplying your bodyweight by 13.

2. What is your fitness goal? Do you want to lose weight or build muscle?

If you want to lose weight, subtract 500 from your RMR. This is the total amount of calories you'll eat on a daily basis.

If you want to build muscle, add 250 to your RMR. This is the total amount of calories you'll need to eat on a daily basis.

Once you know that information, you can move onto the next section.

Setting Up Your Macro Percentages

The first thing we must determine is what percentage of our diet do we want each macronutrient (protein, carb, and fat) to make up? Use the following percentages if your goal is to build muscle:

- Protein: 35% of total calories
- Carbs: 40% of total calories
- Fat: 25% of total calories

And use these percentages if your goal is weight loss:

- Protein: 40% of total calories
- Carbs: 35% of total calories
- Fat: 25% of total calories

At first glance these numbers might not make a lot of sense. Why are we eating so many carbs? Why do you need more protein if you're trying to lose weight as opposed to building muscle?

To address the first question, remember what you learned about carbs from the first chapter. Carbs are very important for making you feel satiated, and carbs are your body's first source of energy. Not only that, but as long as you're creating a caloric deficit, you'll burn fat. Don't buy into all of the low-carb hype!

And to answer the second question, it's more important to have higher amounts of protein when your calories are being restricted. This extra protein will help to prevent muscle loss while you lean down (7). When you're trying to build muscle, your body only needs a certain amount of protein to get the job done.

Anything more than that will not be used to build muscle and will instead be converted into glycogen (8). Sure it would cool if you could simply eat more and more protein and continue to pack on the pounds, but your body doesn't work that way.

Now that you know the total amount of calories you need to eat, and you know the percentage for each macro, we can now determine how many calories of protein, carbs, and fat you'll need to eat. Before we do though, it's important to remember the following:

Number of calories per gram of protein=4
Number of calories per gram of carb=4
Number of calories per gram of fat=9

I'll use myself as an example again:

Resting metabolic rate=2,600 calories

If I want to burn fat:

2,600-500=2,100 daily calories

2,100 x .40= 840 total daily calories from protein
2,100 x .35= 735 total daily calories from carbs
2,100 x .25= 525 total daily calories from fat

You can determine the grams equivalent of these total calorie numbers by doing the following:

840/4=210 grams of protein per day
735/4=183.75 grams of carbs per day
525/9=58.3 grams of fat per day

If I want to build muscle:

2,600+250=2,850 daily calories

2,850 x .35= 997.5 calories from protein
2,850 x .40= 1,140 calories from carbs
2,850 x .25= 712.5 calories from fat

Here are the gram equivalents:

997.5/4=249.4 grams of protein
1,140/4=285 grams of carbs
712.5/9=79.17 grams of fat

If I'm following IIFYM to build muscle, I need to eat roughly 249.4 grams of protein, 285 grams of carbs, and 79.17 grams of fat. So if I eat a 500-calorie cheeseburger that contains 25 grams of fat, 40 grams of protein, and 28.75 grams of carbs, I would subtract those numbers from my daily total:

249.4-40=209.4 grams of protein left to consume
285-28.75=256.25 grams of carbs left to consume
79.17-25=54.17 grams of fat left to consume

For this example, I'm using exact numbers, but the reality is that it'll never be exact and that's ok. I'll explain more about how to actually track your macros and estimate your macros in a later chapter.

Chapter 4: Am I Really Allowed to Eat Whatever I Want?

You may have noticed earlier that I said flexible dieting technically allows you to eat whatever you want as long as it fits within your macro parameters. I say *technically* because while you can eat nothing but junk food and still get results, that's not the most optimal path. Remember, if you're creating a caloric deficit, you'll lose weight regardless of what you eat. A Kansas State professor proved this when he lost over 20 pounds by eating Twinkies (9). To better understand why you shouldn't eat junk food all of the time, we need to ask a classic question—is a calorie a calorie?

Is a Calorie a Calorie?

Yes, a calorie is a calorie just like an inch of wood is the same length as an inch metal. Think about this—what weighs more: a pound of stone or a pound of feathers? They're the same weight! The thing is that it takes way more feathers to reach a pound than it does stone.

The same thing goes for food. 100 calories from broccoli is the same as 100 calories from a candy bar. It's just going to take a lot of broccoli to reach 100 calories. Conversely, it'll take far less of a candy bar to reach those same 100 calories. The real difference between the broccoli and candy bar lies within the macro and micronutrient contents of the foods themselves. The broccoli contains way more vitamins and minerals and will help satisfy you more. On the other hand, the candy bar contains a lot of sugar and empty calories.

What Makes Something Healthy Anyway?

Go around and ask 10 different people what it is that makes a food healthy and you'll likely get 10 different answers. Sure people have a general idea of what foods are healthy vs. not, but it's hard to draw a fine line and say x, y, or z makes a food item unhealthy.

Is it the amount of sugar? The amount of nutrients? What about pasta? Is that healthy if it's whole grain, but unhealthy if it's not? Clearly there are too many variables involved here, and luckily flexible dieting doesn't care about that fine line between healthy and unhealthy. All you need to worry about is eating within your macro parameters.

In fact, this is a common mistake people who're interested in losing weight will make. They'll eliminate all of the "junk food" from their diet and eat nothing but healthy foods. This is a big no-no for a couple of reasons:

1. Eating healthy doesn't guarantee weight loss—a caloric deficit does. Sure healthy foods generally contain fewer calories than junk food, but you can still overeat clean foods.

2. You're not going to go the rest of your life without eating your favorite foods. You'll go insane soon enough, binge eat, and completely ruin your "perfect" wholesome diet.

I'm definitely not for eating healthy all of the time, but I don't advise going crazy with unclean foods either. You must be able to strike a balance between the two. And here's how you'll do exactly that...

The Golden 85% Rule

The golden 85% rule simply states that you eat clean, healthy foods roughly 85% of the time. The other 15% you can eat how you please. This percentage strikes a nice balance between eating junk food and healthy foods. If you eat too much junk food, you'll likely overeat and be low on energy.

However, if you go to the other extreme by eating clean 24/7, you'll drive yourself insane. Eating how you want 15% of the time gives you plenty of wiggle room with flexible dieting. You can eat a small bowl of ice cream every night if you want to. You could enjoy a nice dinner with your friends and family, or do whatever else you want to.

Believing that you can eat junk food all of the time is a big misconception with IIFYM. People who try to abuse the power of flexible dieting will not see lasting results. Sure the diet is flexible, but don't bend it to the point that it breaks. Following the golden 85% rule will help to ensure success with IIFYM.

Chapter 5: How to Actually Track Your Macros

You might be thinking, this sounds great and all, but how do I actually track and measure my macros? This is certainly the most tedious part of IIFYM, but remember what get measured gets managed. You must track and account for the calories you're eating or else you'll have no clue what direction you're heading in.

Simply put, the easiest way to track your macros is to go to the app store, type in IIFYM, and download one of the many apps that will track your macros. Most of the apps cost a couple of dollars, but that's a small price to pay. You can type in the food you're eating and it'll tell you how many calories are contained in the food and how much protein, carbs, and fat it has. Most of the apps even have a bar code scanner where you can take a picture of what you're eating and it'll automatically add the macros towards your daily numbers.

You'll have your phone on you wherever you go, so if you eat at a restaurant, for example, you can track the macros and calories right then and there. If you decide not to use an app, you'll have to track your macros using nutritional labels or by googling the nutritional information online. From there, you'll have to calculate the numbers yourself and record it on a note app or with pen and paper, which is certainly not ideal.

The more inconvenient something is to do, the less likely you are to stick with it. IIFYM is a great nutritional plan, but only if you're able to keep up with it for the long haul. You want to keep things as simple and easy as possible—spend a couple of bucks and indulge in an IIFYM app to take the load off your shoulders. It'll pay for itself many times over.

The other thing you'll need to get is a food scale. You can get one of these on Amazon for around $11. This'll allow you to figure out the number of grams in the foods you're eating and calculate the macros from there.

Once you've been doing IIFYM for a while, you'll eventually start to get a feel for how you need to eat in order to lose weight. You'll know the general macro contents of the meals you regularly eat. You'll be able to do the eyeball test and guess roughly how many calories are in the foods you're eating.

This is a skill that'll come with time. Be patient and don't rush it because that's when you'll start overestimating your calories. Tracking everything as accurately as possible is the key to success with flexible dieting. Be diligent about your measuring especially in the beginning even though it's quite tedious.

It might even take you a couple of weeks to get used to measuring and recording everything that you eat and drink. Be patient with yourself if it takes a few weeks for you to start seeing results. You'll get better and better with the process as time goes on. Nobody is a master at something the first time they do it.

One common question people have with IIFYM is how close do I have to be with my macro percentages and calories? The reality is that you'll never be 100% spot on accurate with your numbers. Using the example from earlier, you'll never eat exactly 79.17 grams of fat each day and that's ok. You'll want to aim to be within 5-10% of what I recommend. For example, one day you might intake 30% of your diet from fat and only 30% from protein. It's not worth the extra stress of getting every little number exactly right—you'll drive yourself nuts. You want to generally be as consistent and accurate as you possibly can.

Chapter 6: The Importance of Exercise

IIFYM is a great nutritional strategy that can help you build muscle or burn fat. However, if you want to build your best physique possible, you must incorporate exercise into your regimen as well, more specifically resistance training. Lifting weights is what will stimulate your muscles to grow, and it's how you'll build a lean and muscular look.

Sure you can lean down using flexible dieting, but something won't look quite right when you reach your end goal. You'll end up looking flat, skinny, and weak if you only diet. On the other hand, if you do resistance training while you lose weight, you'll end up looking fit and defined. The cool thing is that you only need to lift weights 2-3 times per week in order to maintain and build new muscle mass (10).

The workout routine I'll be providing to you contains two different workouts—A and B. You'll simply alternate between workout A and workout B every time you go to the gym. Here's an example of how to set up your gym schedule depending on how many days per week you want to workout:

If you want to workout 2 times per week:

Monday: Off
Tuesday: Workout A
Wednesday: Off
Thursday: Off
Friday: Workout B

Saturday: Off
Sunday: Off

If you want to workout 3 times per week:

Monday: Workout A
Tuesday: Off
Wednesday: Workout B
Thursday: Off
Friday: Workout A
Saturday: Off
Sunday: Off

Following Monday: Workout B

If you want to workout 4 times per week:

Monday: Workout A
Tuesday: Workout B
Wednesday: Off
Thursday: Workout A
Friday: Workout B
Saturday: Off
Sunday: Off

Here are the workouts:

Workout A: Chest, Shoulders, and Triceps

- Incline Barbell Bench Press- 3 sets of 6 reps 3 min rest

  btw (between) sets

- Seated DB Military Press- 3 sets of 6 reps 3 min rest

  btw sets

- DB Skull Crushers- 3 sets of 8 reps 90 sec rest btw sets

- Standing DB Lateral Raises- 3 sets of 10 reps 1 min rest btw sets

- Bent Lateral Raises- 3 sets of 12 reps 1 min rest btw sets

Workout B: Back, Legs, and Biceps

- Weighted Pull-Ups (replace with lat-pulldown if unable to do pull-ups)- 3 sets of 6 reps

- Bulgarian Split Squats- 3 sets of 8 reps (per leg) 2 min rest btw sets

- Incline DB Curls- 3 sets of 8 reps 90 sec rest btw sets

- Bent Over Rows- 3 sets of 8 reps 2 min rest btw sets

- Hammer Curls- 3 sets of 10 reps 1 min rest btw sets

This is a good workout to do regardless of whether or not you want to build muscle or burn fat. Many people try to change up their workout and do higher reps when trying to burn fat. Many people think that higher reps burn fat and lower reps build muscle, but that is a big myth. All rep ranges build muscle; they stimulate a different type of hypertrophy— sarcoplasmic vs myofibrillar.

Sure higher reps might burn a few extra calories, which might indirectly lead to fat loss, but don't rely on it. The easiest way to think about it is to use your workouts to help you build muscle, and use your diet to help you control your calories for fat loss.

In addition to weight training, you can also do cardio. However, only doing cardio with flexible dieting will still leave you looking flat and skinny. Do cardio with your weight training for a complete fitness routine. The cool thing about cardio is that it'll either give you more leeway with your IIFYM diet, or you'll lean down that much faster. Here's the cardio routine you should do 2-3 times per week if your goal is fat loss:

Part 1: High Intensity Interval Training (HIIT)

Alternate between a high intensity and a low intensity for 15-30 minutes on your choice of cardio machine. Here's an example on a treadmill:

- Run at 7.5 mph for 1 minute
- Walk at 3.5 mph for 1 minute
- Repeat for 10-15 minutes

Part 2: Steady State Cardio (Done immediately after HIIT)

Example on a treadmill: Walk at a constant pace of 3.5-4 mph for 10-15 minutes

Note: If you need to adjust the intensity of the HIIT then do so. You can alter the run walk ratios (i.e. run for 30 seconds and walk for 1.5 minutes), or you can decrease the intensity of each run (i.e. run at 6 mph instead of 7.5). And if what I prescribed is too easy then ramp up the intensity accordingly.

The secret to the effectiveness of this workout lies in the fact that we're combining intense cardio with slow, steady state cardio. Most people will do one or the other, but not both in the same cardio session. The intense cardio will release free fatty acids into the bloodstream, and then the steady state cardio will burn them off! If you only did the HIIT, your body would reabsorb the released fatty acids. That's why you want to combine both for maximum efficiency.

Chapter 7: How to Properly Set and Achieve Your Fitness Goals

Again, I get that this is a book about flexible dieting, but I don't want you to learn solely about that topic. I want to give you a complete fitness routine- one you can easily do and maintain for the rest of your life.

I want to give you all of the tools necessary for you to be successful with fitness. Doing things like training in the gym and setting goals are how you'll separate yourself from people who are only willing to diet to get fit. Research does show that writing down your goals will make you more likely to achieve them as opposed to keeping them in your head (11). Sadly only 3% of people write down their goals regularly (12).

5 Reasons Why You Should Write Your Goals

Reason #1: Writing down your goals makes what you want real.

You've clarified exactly what you want and you can work backwards from there until you achieve it.

Reason #2: More likely to stick to it.

You'll be much less likely to give up if you wrote it down and made a commitment to yourself (and others).

Reason #3: The law of attraction

Basically, what you think about the most is what you'll attract into your life. By writing your goals, you'll keep them at the front of your mind making it more likely to happen.

Reason #4: More likely to actually achieve your goal

Yes, there is evidence to show that you're more likely to achieve your goal by writing it down (13).

Reason #5: Gives focus to your day

You can wake up each morning knowing exactly what it is that you need to do for the day.

8 Tips to Properly Write Your Goals and See Success

Tip #1: Write Them With Pen and Paper
You learn better when you write things down as opposed to typing (14). You can of course keep another list of your goals on your computer if you like. Just remember though, it'll stick in your head better when you write them down.

Tip #2: Write Your Goals Every Day

Writing your goals every day helps you keep them at the front of your mind. Best practice is to write them soon after waking and before going to bed. This way your goals are always the first and last thing on your mind.

Tip #3: Set a Deadline

A goal without a deadline is kinda like a wish—if it happens one day then great, if not then oh well. When you set a concrete deadline to your goal, it makes it very real. Now you know how long you have to reach your goal and you can work backwards from there. What if you don't achieve your goal by the set deadline? Don't sweat it, and simply set a new deadline. With certain goals, it'll be hard to judge a realistic timeframe so take your best guess.

Tip #4: Write Them in the Present Tense

When you write your goals, you want to write them in the present tense as if you've already achieved them. The main reason for this is because our subconscious mind only recognizes the present tense and not what happened or is going to happen. For example, don't say, "I will weigh 150 pounds by July 15, 2017." Instead it's better to make it present, "I weigh 150 pounds by July 15, 2017."

Tip #5: Set as Many Goals as You Like

Another common question about goal setting is, "How many goals should I set?"
There isn't a limit. The more goals you set the better. Don't limit yourself to setting one goal. Set 10 goals if that's what you want to achieve.

Tip #6: Set Goals for all Areas of Life

Also don't limit yourself to setting exclusively fitness goals. While it's important, it's not everything. You could set goals that relate to your career, family, or personal improvement as well. For example:

Family: Incorporate a family game night once per week by May 25, 2017.
Career: I learn more about [blank] and become a better [blank] by June 1,2017.
Personal Improvement: I watch only 30 minutes of T.V. a day by July 30,2017.

Tip #7: Focus on the Process Not Just the Outcome

Outcome goals are great because they're like the top of a mountain—that's where you want to go. Process goals, on the other hand, are the things that you're going to do to be able to reach the top of the mountain. Here's an example:

Outcome Goal: I weigh 165 pounds by June 1, 2017.
Process Goals: Drink only water.
                  Go to the gym 3 times per week.
                  Eat more fruits and vegetables.

Process goals are great because they give you guidance on what to do in your day-to-day life. If you don't end up achieving your outcome goal, you can look back at your process goals and adjust them. Conversely, if you set an outcome goal and didn't achieve it, you wouldn't know why you failed or what to do differently. In the example above, let's say June 1st rolls around and you're nowhere close to 165 pounds.

The first thing to do is to ask yourself if you actually executed on the process goals. If you did, then you need to reassess your process. For example, you might need to eat sweets and other such foods in moderation. I recommend having at least 3 process goals for each outcome goal that you have.

Side Note: Make sure that you write down your process goals in addition to your outcome goals.

Tip #8: Write Your Goals on Notecards

In addition to writing your goals on notebook paper everyday, keep your goals on notecards as well. Then stick it in your wallet, purse, car, or wherever else you'll be and look at them throughout the day. This way you'll keep your goals at the front of your mind all day long. It'll also help to keep you motivated and narrow your focus down to the most important task.

Side Note: You don't have to rewrite your goals on the notecards everyday, just once will do.

Tip #9: Share Your Goals With Others

Sharing and being open with people is hard. What will others think of your goals? What will they say if you fail? However, if you really want something bad enough, you'll share your goals with as many people as possible. The reason why is because as humans, we want to be consistent with what we say.

In an experiment conducted in 1987 (15), a social scientist went around asking potential voters the day before the election if they were going to vote and why/why not. Of the people asked, 100% said yes they would vote. On the election, 86.7% of those people asked did vote compared to only 61.5% who weren't asked.
If you start sharing your goals and ambitions with others, you'll want to be congruent with what you say to them. You won't want to let them down. You'll be held accountable and do what it takes to get the job done. If you don't share your goals, then what happens if you don't achieve them? Absolutely nothing. And that can be a big problem if you're ready for a change in your life.

Chapter 8: 42 Macro Recipes

Rainbow Trout

Ingredients:

- 2 Rainbow trout fillets
- 1 tbsp. olive oil
- 1 tbsp. black pepper

Directions:

1. Preheat boiler to 500 degrees F.
2. Put the fillets on boiler pan.
3. Place fish in boiler, leaving door ajar enough to keep heat source on constantly.
4. Set timer for 4 minutes.
5. Take out and serve.

Number of servings: 2

Macros:

Total calories: 282.3

Protein: 33.1 g
Carbs: 2.1 g
Fat: 15.2 g

*Recipe courtesy of COLLINSLG

Balsamic Chicken

Ingredients:

- 1 Chicken breast
- 4 tbsp. balsamic vinegar
- 2 tsp. chopped garlic
- 1 tsp. olive oil
- Salt and pepper for taste

Directions:

1. Cut chicken breast in thin 2-inch strips.
2. Chop garlic.
3. Heat oil in a pan and add garlic. Sauté until golden.
4. Add chicken and stir well.
5. Add balsamic vinegar and salt and pepper.
6. Reduce heat to medium and let excess water evaporate.
7. Keep stirring and make sure all the water dries up and the chicken is well coated with balsamic vinegar.
8. Serve when thoroughly cooked.

Number of servings: 1

Macros:

Total calories: 166.5

Protein: 16.8 g
Carbs: 9.9 g
Fat: 5.4 g

*Recipe courtesy of JASSLAMBA

Tuna Salad

Ingredients:

- 6 oz. of tuna
- ½ cup of 1% cottage cheese
- ½ large tomato
- 1.5 cups shredded romaine lettuce
- ¼ cup onion

Directions:

1. Mix tuna with cottage cheese.
2. Cut up lettuce and tomatoes.
3. Add all of the ingredients into a bowl and mix.
4. Serve and enjoy!

Number of servings: 1

Macros:

Total calories: 275.4

Protein: 49.1 g
Carbs: 12.7 g
Fat: 2.7 g

*Recipe courtesy of STEFERFLY7

Protein Crepes

Ingredients:

- ½ cup egg whites
- 1 scoop of protein powder
- Touch of water

Directions:

1. Blend water and protein powder briefly.
2. Combine mixture with egg whites.
3. Pour 1/3 of mixture in a nonstick pan.
4. Cook until bubbles form.
5. Flip and cook for 10 more seconds.
6. Repeat until all of the mixture is cooked.

Number of servings: 1

Marcos:

Total calories: 158.0

Protein: 31.4 g
Carbs: 3.0 g
Fat: 2.4 g

Recipe courtesy of MAKOTO1

Cinnamon Greek Yogurt

Ingredients:

- 6 oz. plain Greek yogurt
- 1 tsp. ground cinnamon
- 1 packet Truvia

Directions:

1. Add cinnamon and Truvia to yogurt and mix in small bowl.

Number of servings: 1

Macros:

Total calories: 106.0

Protein: 14.1 g
Carbs: 14.8
Fat: .1 g

*Recipe courtesy of JEANNESERENITY

Protein Powder Pancakes

Ingredients:

- ½ cup oats
- ½ cup hot water
- 1 scoop protein powder
- ¼ cup egg whites
- ¼ tsp. ground cinnamon

Directions:

2. Mix oats with hot water.
3. Stir and let sit for a couple of minutes until fluffy.
4. Mix protein powder with the egg whites and then mix with oats.
5. Add in cinnamon and fry on griddle.

Number of servings: 4

Macros:

Total calories (per serving): 77.1

Protein: 8.9 g
Carbs: 7.8 g
Fat: .8g

*Recipe courtesy of FITGIRL15

Protein Shake

Ingredients:

- ¾ cup frozen strawberries
- 1 scoop vanilla protein powder
- ¾ cup of water
- 1 tbsp. ground flax seed
- 1 ¼ cup ice

Directions:

1. Add ingredients to blender.
2. Blend for desired consistency.

Number of servings: 1

Macros:

Total calories: 199.1

Protein: 21.0 g
Carbs: 18.2 g
Fat: 4.9 g

*Recipe courtesy of MY_BEST_LIFE

Protein Salad

Ingredients:

- 1 cup garbanzo beans
- 1 cup diced cucumber
- ½ cup carrots
- ½ red bell pepper
- 2 onions
- ¼ cup sunflower seeds
- 1/8 cup parsley
- 1 cup of wheat

Dressing ingredients:

- 1 cup whey
- 1 cup cottage cheese
- 1 tbsp. apple cider vinegar
- 1 tsp. crushed garlic
- 1 tsp. sea salt
- 1 tsp. black pepper

Directions:

1. Mix together dressing ingredients until consistent.
2. Combine salad ingredients and pour dressing over.

Number of servings: 4

Macros (per serving):

Total calories: 348.3

Protein: 20.2 g
Carbs: 64.8 g
Fat: 2.9 g

*Recipe courtesy of WANNABTHNAGN29

Protein Bars

Ingredients:

- 1 scoop chocolate protein powder
- 1 tbsp. cocoa powder
- 1/3 cup Splenda
- 1 cup oats
- 4 egg whites
- ½ cup applesauce
- ¼ tsp. vanilla extract
- 1 tbsp. peanut butter

Directions:

1. Preheat oven to 350 degrees F.
2. Mix egg whites and uncooked oatmeal.
3. Add remaining ingredients.
4. Spread mixture in an even layer over bottom layer of dish.
5. Bake for 15-20 minutes.

Number of servings: 9

Macros (per serving):

Total calories: 71.5

Protein: 6.4g
Carbs: 9.8g
Fat: 1.5g

*Recipe courtesy of CORNPOPGIRL

Blueberry Protein Muffins

Ingredients:

- 2 cup uncooked oat bran
- ¼ cup brown sugar
- 2 tsp. baking powder
- 1 scoop vanilla protein powder
- ¼ cup skim milk
- 1 cup plain greek yogurt
- 2 large egg whites
- 2 tbsp. canola oil
- ½ cup blueberries

Directions:

1. Preheat oven to 425 degrees F.
2. Combine dry ingredients in a bowl.
3. Combine wet ingredients in separate bowl and add to dry mix.
4. Mix until moistened.
5. Add in blueberries.
6. Fill in muffin cups until close to full.
7. Bake for 20 minutes.

Number of Servings: 12

Macros (per serving):

Total calories: 165.9

Protein: 8.8g
Carbs: 165.9 g
Fat: 3.8 g

*Recipe courtesy of SARAH_45

Peanut Butter Squares

Ingredients:

- 32.4 g of natural crunchy peanut butter
- 5 scoops of your choice of protein powder
- 3.24 g of brown linseeds
- ½ cup of water

Directions:

1. Mix protein powder and linseeds with peanut butter until a crumply dough forms.
2. Slowly add water to form a thick paste.
3. Mold paste into app. 6.5x6.5 cm cookies and seal in plastic wrap.
4. Refrigerate and enjoy!

Number of servings: 10

Macros (per serving):

Total calories: 361.5

Protein: 23.2 g
Carbs: 9.6 g
Fat: 25.7 g

*Recipe courtesy of TANIA83

Baked Potato Soup

Ingredients:

- 6 large potatoes
- 3 large carrots
- 3 celery stalks
- 2 onions
- 4 chicken bouillon cubes
- 6 cups of water

Directions:

1. Combine all ingredients into a large crock pot. Cook on low for 8-10 hours and serve.

Number of servings: 12

Macros (per serving):

Total calories: 170.7

Protein: 5.9 g
Carbs: 36.7 g
Fat: .4 g

*Recipe courtesy of JHENGESH

Sweet Potato Fries

Ingredients:

- 2 large sweet potatoes
- 1/8 cup extra virgin olive oil
- 5 tbsp. Splenda
- 1 tbsp. ground cinnamon
- 2 tbsp. salt

Directions:

1. Cut sweet potatoes into thin strips.
2. Preheat oven to 425 degrees F.
3. Combine Splenda, cinnamon, and salt in a small bowl.
4. Arrange sweet potatoes on cookie sheet in one layer.
5. Drizzle with olive oil.
6. Sprinkle with Splenda mixture.
7. Bake for 30 minutes and enjoy!

Number of servings: 3

Macros (per serving):

Total calories: 177.2

Protein: 1.5g
Carbs: 22.6 g
Fat: 9.7 g

*Recipe courtesy of EVELEZ

Chicken Tacos

Ingredients:

- 24 oz. of chicken
- 1 cup chopped onions
- 1 cup diced tomatoes
- 3 oz. spinach leaves
- ½ cup of salsa
- 1 cup shredded cheese
- 1 packet of taco seasoning
- ¾ cup of water

Directions:

1. Cut up chicken into small pieces.
2. Chop onions into fine pieces.
3. Cook chicken and onions in skillet on medium heat.
4. Add taco seasoning and water to chicken and onions.
5. Reduce heat and let the sauce stand for thickness.
6. Add chicken and sides for filling

Number of servings: 5

Macros (per serving):

Total calories: 449.9

Protein: 44.4 g
Carbs: 37.4 g
Fat: 11.5 g

*Recipe courtesy of JONSMASH

Breakfast Tacos

Ingredients:

- 4 small flour tortillas
- 3 eggs
- 2 cups diced potatoes
- ½ cup of cheese
- Salt and pepper to taste

Directions:

1. Sauté potatoes in oil and thoroughly cook for 4-5 minutes.
2. Whisk eggs in small bowl with a tablespoon of water.
3. Add eggs to potatoes and scramble together.
4. Remove from heat and add in cheese.
5. Place in tortillas and enjoy!

Number of servings: 4

Macros (per serving):

Total calories: 311.0

Protein: 14.6 g
Carbs: 25.2 g
Fat: 16.8 g

*Recipe courtesy of ROSABELLE61

Spaghetti and Turkey Meat

Ingredients:

- 1 pound of lean turkey meat
- ½ large onion
- 10 cloves of garlic
- 8 oz. sliced mushrooms
- 1 jar of tomato sauce
- 2 boxes of spaghetti

Directions:

1. Brown turkey meat.
2. Add onion, garlic, and mushrooms to turkey meat.
3. Boil spaghetti.
4. Add tomato sauce.
5. Add meat combination and enjoy.

Number of servings: 14

Macros (per serving):

Total calories: 282.2

Protein: 14.1 g
Carbs: 50.0 g
Fat: 5.1 g

*Recipe courtesy of 73STRAWBERRIES

Tomato Chicken Pasta

Ingredients:

- 10 strands of angel hair pasta
- 2 medium carrots
- 1 tbsp. of chopped onion
- 1 chopped cauliflower
- 3 tbsp. of tomatoes
- 3 oz. of chicken breast

Directions:

1. Cook pasta and set aside.
2. Sauté carrots, onion, and cauliflower on low heat with oil.
3. Add in chicken and tomatoes.
4. Stir the mixture up and add in pasta.
5. Continue to stir mixture and cook on low heat until thoroughly cooked.

Number of servings: 1

Macros:

Total calories: 222.7

Protein: 26.2 g
Carbs: 26.6 g
Fat: 2.2 g

*Recipe courtesy of GREENIETWO

Chicken Alfredo

Ingredients:

- 1 pound of pasta
- ½ cup of butter
- 1 pound of chicken breasts
- 2- 16oz containers of ricotta cheese
- 1 pint of heavy cream
- 1 cup of Parmesan cheese

Directions:

1. Boil a large pot of water.
2. Add pasta and cook for 10 minutes.
3. Drain out the water.
4. Melt 2 tablespoons of butter in large skillet on medium heat.
5. Sauté chicken until thoroughly cooked.
6. Combine ricotta cheese, cream, and Parmesan cheese and remaining butter in a saucepan.
7. Cook mixture on medium heat for about 10 minutes.
8. Add in pasta and chicken and continue cooking until thoroughly done.

Number of servings: 8

Macros (per serving):

Total calories: 770.2

Protein: 26.4 g
Carbs: 19.3 g
Fat: 66.1 g

*Recipe courtesy of RUSSIANTM

Cottage Cheese Fruit Bowl

Ingredients:

- 1 cup of cottage cheese
- 1 tbsp. of honey
- 1 medium sized apricot
- 1 handful of cherries
- ½ cup of mango
- ¼ cup of granola

Directions:

1. Blend cottage cheese and honey.
2. Sprinkle granola onto cottage cheese in a bowl.
3. Cut fruit into small pieces.
4. Place fruit on top of cottage cheese and enjoy.

Number of servings: 1

Macros:

Total calories: 521.4

Protein: 37.1 g
Carbs: 68.3 g
Fat: 12.3 g

*Recipe courtesy HEALTHBLOGGER

Cottage Cheese Scramble

Ingredients:

- 1/3 cup instant dry milk
- ¼ cup of water
- 3 eggs
- ½ cup cottage cheese
- ½ tsp salt
- 2 tbsp. of butter

Directions:

1. Blend together all of the ingredients minus the butter.
2. Melt the butter in a skillet.
3. Add egg mixture to skillet and cook on low heat and enjoy!

Number of servings: 3

Macros (per serving):

Total calories: 169.1

Protein: 14.1 g
Carbs: 6.0 g
Fat: 9.6 g

*Recipe courtesy of CALL-ME

Stuffed Green Peppers

Ingredients:

- 4 large green peppers
- ½ cup onions
- 1 cup mushrooms
- 1 tbsp. olive oil
- 1 tsp. fresh thyme leaves
- 1 tsp. chopped garlic
- 1 tsp. sun dried tomatoes
- 1 lb. ground beef
- 1 cup brown rice
- 28 oz. diced tomatoes
- 3 oz. tomato paste
- 4 tbsp. parmesan cheese

Directions:

1. Preheat oven to 375 degrees F.
2. Cook rice according to package directions.
3. Heat olive oil in skillet and add onions, mushrooms, garlic, sun dried tomatoes, thyme, and beef.
4. Add one cup of rice, can of tomatoes and tomato paste.
5. Cut the tops of the bell peppers off and add in the stuffing.
6. Cook for 30 minutes.
7. Add parmesan cheese and cook for an additional 5 minutes.

Number of servings: 4

Macros (per serving):

Total calories: 480.2

Protein: 29.2 g

Carbs: 36.4 g
Fat: 25.4 g

*Recipe courtesy of R_HAMILTON

Garlic Mashed Potatoes

Ingredients:

- 1 lb. of potatoes
- 1 cup skim milk
- 6 large cloves of garlic
- ½ teaspoon white pepper

Directions:

1. Cook potatoes in boiling water for 25 minutes.
2. Simmer garlic and pepper in milk until garlic is soft.
3. Add milk and garlic mixture to potatoes.
4. Beat potatoes with electric mixer on low speed until smooth.

Number of servings: 4

Macros (per serving):

Total calories: 167.6

Protein: 4.6 g
Carbs: 29.2 g
Fat: 4.0 g

*Recipe courtesy of WHITEBOY23

Cauliflower Soup

Ingredients:

- 1 head of cabbage
- 1 head of cauliflower
- 6- 14.5 oz. cans low sodium chicken broth
- ¼ cup blue cheese crumbles

Directions:

1. Chop cabbage and cauliflower and place in large pot.
2. Add in enough chicken broth to cover cabbage and cauliflower.
3. Cover pot and cook for 60-90 minutes.
4. Remove from heat and add in cheese and pepper.
5. Puree in blender.

Number of servings: 18

Macros (per serving):

Total calories 40.8

Protein: 3.7 g
Carbs: 6.1 g
Fat: .9 g

*Recipe courtesy of: KAT.COURTNEY

High Protein Waffles

Ingredients:

- ¾ scoop vanilla protein powder
- 1 egg
- 1/3 tsp. baking powder
- 2 tbsp. water
- 1 tsp. oil

Directions:

1. Blend ingredients together until smooth.
2. Grease waffle maker.
3. Add mixture to griddle and cook like normal waffle.

Number of servings: 1

Macros:

Total calories: 186.6

Protein: 17.4 g
Carbs: 6.0 g
Fat: 10.4 g

*Recipe courtesy of FLUFFY22801

High Protein Chocolate Granola

Ingredients:

- 6 cups rolled oats
- 1 cup sliced almonds
- ½ cup non-fat dry milk powder
- 2 scoops chocolate protein powder
- ¼ cup brown rice syrup
- 1 tbsp. oil
- ½ tbsp. stevia extract
- ½ cup water
- ¼ cup mini chocolate chips

Directions:

1. Preheat oven to 250 degrees F.
2. Combine oats, protein powder, milk, milk powder, and almonds in a large bowl and mix the ingredients well.
3. Mix wet ingredients (water, oil, brown rice syrup, and stevia) in a small bowl.
4. Spread in a pan and bake in oven.
5. Remove from oven and add in chocolate chips.

Number of servings: 24

Macros (per serving):

Total calories: 157.1

Protein: 7.2 g
Carbs: 21.6 g
Fat: 5.1 g

*Recipe courtesy of SELVAGEEDGE

High Protein Cookies

Ingredients:

- 4 tsp. butter substitute
- 2 scoops chocolate protein powder
- 8 tsp. of Splenda
- 3 tsp. of water

Directions:

1. In a bowl, microwave butter for 20 seconds.
2. Add in protein powder and Splenda to bowl.
3. Gradually add water to mixture, until you can form the mixture in a ball.
4. Heat ball mixture in microwave for 15-30 seconds.

Number of servings: 4

Macros (per serving):

Total calories: 100

Protein: 13.5 g
Carbs: 4.5 g
Fat 3.0 g

*Recipe courtesy of SADIE78

High Protein, Low Carb Pumpkin Bread

Ingredients:

- 1/4 tsp. ground cloves
- 1/2 tsp. ground nutmeg
- 1 tsp. baking soda
- 1/4 cup of oats
- 100 grams almond flour
- 1/4 cup applesauce
- 3 tsp. baking powder
- 50 grams pecans
- 0.8 cup of stevia
- 8 tbsp. egg whites
- 4 tsp. cinnamon
- ½ cup Pumpkin-Libby's pumpkin
- 30 grams oat bran cereal
- 2 servings whey protein powder
- 20 grams flaxseed

Directions:

1. Preheat oven to 325 degrees F.
2. Mix all of the dry ingredients in a bowl.
3. Mix wet ingredients together in a separate bowl.
4. Fix two large loaf pans.
5. Combine the wet mixture with the dry mixture.
6. Pour combined mixture into fixed pans and bake for 25 minutes.
7. Remove and let it cool for 5-10 minutes.

Number of servings: 16

Macros (per serving):

Total calories: 127.1

Protein: 9.3 g
Carbs: 10.8 g
Fat: 6.2 g

*Recipe courtesy of DRMOM7310

Lemon Garlic Tilapia

Ingredients:

- 4 tilapia fillets
- 3 tbsp. lemon juice
- 1 garlic clove
- 1 tsp. dried parsley flakes
- Salt, pepper, and garlic powder to taste

Directions:

1. Preheat oven to 375 degrees F.
2. Put tilapia fillets in baking dish.
3. Pour lemon juice over fillets.
4. Add in desired salt, pepper, and garlic powder.
5. Bake tilapia for around 30 minutes.

Number of servings: 4

Macros (per serving):

Total calories: 116.7

Protein: 22.8 g
Carbs: 2.9 g
Fat: 1.9 g

*Recipe courtesy of SADIE78

Jambalaya

Ingredients:

- 4 chicken breasts
- 6 Italian sausages
- 1 large chopped onion
- ¾ cup chopped green pepper
- 2 jalapeno peppers
- 2 garlic cloves
- 1 tbsp. canola oil
- 2 cans of diced tomatoes
- 1 small can tomato paste
- ½ cup of water
- 1 tsp. dried thyme
- ½ tsp. salt
- ¼ tsp. pepper
- 1/8 cayenne pepper
- 1 lb. uncooked shrimp
- 2 cups brown rice

Directions:

1. Chop up chicken into 1 inch slices.
2. Chop up sausage.
3. Sauté chicken, sausage, onion, green pepper, jalapenos, and garlic in oil until chicken is thoroughly cooked.
4. Throw in tomatoes, salt, pepper, and cayenne and bring to boil.
5. Simmer for 15 minutes and add shrimp.
6. Simmer for another 8 minutes.
7. Stir in rice.

Number of servings: 6

Macros (per serving):

Total calories: 261.5

Protein: 27.9 g
Carbs: 25.7 g
Fat: 5.3 g

*Recipe courtesy of SADIE78

Vegetable and Seafood Soup

Ingredients:

- 12 oz. salmon
- 12 oz. scallops
- 2 lb. of shrimp
- 5 diced medium carrots
- 6 stalks of celery
- 2 diced green peppers
- 1 diced onion
- 5 sliced garlic clove
- 2 cups zucchini
- 28 oz. canned tomatoes
- 4 cups of chicken broth
- 6 cups of water
- 1/2 tsp. thyme
- 1/2 tsp. basil
- 1 tsp. crushed red pepper
- 1 tbsp. parsley
- 2 tbsp. olive oil

Directions:

1. Dice vegetables and put 2 tbsp. of olive oil in heated pot.
2. Add in onion, garlic, bell pepper, carrots, celery, zucchini and cook for 6 minutes.
3. Add in basil, thyme, crushed pepper, crushed bay leaves, salmon, scallops, diced canned tomatoes, chicken broth, and water.
4. Bring to boil and cook for additional 12 minutes.
5. Season with salt and cook for another 10 minutes on low heat.
6. Add in parsley and cook for 5 more minutes and enjoy.

Number of servings: 24

Macros (per serving):

Total calories: 120.0

Protein: 16.9 g
Carbs: 5.8 g
Fat: 3.2 g

*Recipe courtesy of ANUME1109
Protein Brownies

Ingredients:

- 4 oz. chocolate
- 2.2 oz. flour
- 2 oz. soy flour
- 6 tbsp. protein powder
- 2 tbsp. ground flaxseed
- ¼ tsp baking powder
- ½ tsp salt
- 3 oz. cocoa powder
- 10 oz. tofu
- 3 oz. granulated sugar
- 7 oz. brown sugar
- 2 tsp. vanilla
- ¼ cup canola oil
- ½ cup soymilk
- 2 oz. mini chocolate chips

Directions:

1. Preheat oven to 350 degrees F.

2. Melt chocolate in small bowl in microwave and place to the side.
3. In a separate bowl, whisk the flours, protein powder, flaxseed, baking powder, salt, and cocoa.
4. Puree tofu, granulated sugar, and brown sugar until smooth.
5. Add in melted chocolate, vanilla, canola oil, and soymilk to processor and blend until smooth.
6. Add dry mixture to current ingredients in processor and pulse as needed.
7. Add in mini chocolate chips and pulse shortly.
8. Pour mixture into a pan.
9. Bake for 25 minutes and cool for 5-10 minutes.

Number of servings: 24

Macros (per serving):

Total calories: 172.5

Protein: 5.8 g
Carbs: 27.1 g
Fat 6.7 g

*Recipe courtesy of JO_JO_BA

Salsa Turkey Burgers

Ingredients:

- 1 lb. ground turkey meat
- 1/3 cup seasoned bread crumbs
- 4 tbsp. chunky salsa
- Salt and pepper to taste.
- Add topping as desired.

Directions:

1. Combine all ingredients until well mixed.
2. Add salt and pepper to taste.
3. Divide into 4 patties.
4. Cook in frying pan over medium for around 10 minutes and flip patties roughly halfway through.

Number of servings: 4

Macros (per serving):

Total calories: 161.8

Protein: 29.4 g
Carbs: 7.6 g
Fat: 1.5 g

*Recipe courtesy of JIMINNYC

Koshari

Ingredients:

- 1 cup dry green lentils
- 1 cup of pasta
- 1 cup of brown rice
- 2 cups of tomato sauce
- 1 large chopped onion
- 2 chopped cloves of garlic
- 1 chopped green bell pepper
- 2 tbsp. olive oil
- 4 oz. chicken tenders

Directions:

1. Put lentils and pasta in saucepan and boil, simmer on low for 25 minutes.
2. Cook rice in 2 cups of water separately while lentils are cooking.
3. Combine lentils, rice, and macaroni in large pot.
4. Sauté onions, bell pepper, and garlic with olive oil until brown.
5. Add chicken tenders and tomato sauce to the onions and garlic and cook until bubbles form.
6. Pour sauce over original mixture and enjoy!

Number of servings: 8

Macros (per serving):

Total calories: 208.8

Protein: 10.8 g
Carbs: 33.4 g
Fat: 4.2 g

*Recipe courtesy of NICOLETTEDIMON

High Protein Minestrone

Ingredients:

- 1 tbsp. olive oil
- ½ cup chopped onions
- 1 clove of garlic
- 1 can of diced tomatoes
- 1 ½ cups of vegetable broth
- 1 tbsp. tomato paste
- 1 can of kidney beans
- 1 can of black beans
- 16 oz. bag of frozen vegetables
- Salt and pepper to taste

Directions:

1. Sauté onion and garlic in saucepan with oil.
2. Add in the can of diced tomatoes and vegetable broth.
3. Add in beans and frozen vegetables.
4. Bring to boil and simmer for 30 minutes.

Number of servings: 4

Macros (per serving):

Total calories: 362.6

Protein: 19.1 g
Carbs: 65.6 g
Fat: 4.8 g

*Recipe courtesy of TONYNE

High Protein Chocolate Pudding

Ingredients:

- 7.5 oz. tofu
- 1/3 cups unsweetened cocoa
- ¾ cups stevia
- 6 oz. vanilla greek yogurt
- 1 tsp. vanilla
- cinnamon to taste

Directions:

1. Chop tofu into pieces.
2. Place all ingredients in food processor and blend until smooth.
3. Place in plastic container and refrigerate for 2 hours.

Number of servings: 4

Macros (per serving):

Total calories: 118.5

Protein: 11.4 g
Carbs: 13.8 g
Fat: 4.7 g

*Recipe courtesy of SHORTPUTTS

Low Carb/High Protein Pizza

Ingredients:

- 2 cans of cream cheese
- 2 eggs
- 1 cup parmesan cheese
- 2 tbsp. garlic
- 1 can tomato paste
- 2 tbsp. oregano
- 2 tbsp. basil
- 1 tsp. salt
- Water as needed

Directions:

1. Mix cream cheese, eggs, and parmesan cheese together until smooth.
2. Preheat oven to 350 degrees F.
3. Pour mix on pan and spread evenly.
4. Put pan in oven for 45 minutes.
5. Let crust cool for 10 minutes.
6. Pour tomato paste into a bowl.
7. Add oregano, basil, salt, garlic, and add necessary water for desired thickness.
8. Once sauce is made, pour and spread evenly over the cooled crust.
9. Put desired toppings on sauce.
10. Place pizza back in the oven for 30 minutes.
11. Let it cool for 5-10 minutes and enjoy!

Number of servings: 8

Macros (per serving):

Total calories: 213.2

Protein: 13.1 g

Carbs: 6.0 g
Fat: 15.4 g

*Recipe courtesy of NATIVITY4ME

Protein Shake to Build Muscle Mass

Ingredients:

- ½ cup of milk
- ½ cup of oats
- ½ cup of water
- 2 tbsp. peanut butter
- 1 large banana
- 4 scoops of protein powder

Directions:

1. Put all ingredients in blender and blend on high until smooth.

Number of servings: 2

Macros (per serving):

Total calories: 443.9

Protein: 36.7 g
Carbs: 61.2 g
Fat: 13.2 g

*Recipe courtesy of BRUTALCHICK

Chicken Cacciatore

Ingredients:

- 4 chicken breasts chopped up
- 2 diced green peppers
- 4 diced onions
- 2 cans stewed tomatoes mashed up
- 1 large can of mushroom pieces
- 2 tbsp. olive oil
- garlic powder and salt to taste
- 1 lb. of spaghetti noodles
- Grated parmesan cheese to taste

Directions:

1. Brown chicken in oil.
2. Separately brown onions and peppers.
3. Season with herbs, tomatoes, and mushrooms.
4. Simmer mixture for 15 minutes.
5. Add in chicken and cook for 45 minutes.
6. Cook spaghetti in pot and drain.
7. Add chicken mixture to spaghetti and top with Parmesan cheese.

Number of servings: 5

Macros (per serving): 345.6

Total calories: 345.6

Protein: 37.7 g
Carbs: 32.5 g
Fat: 7.6 g

*Recipe courtesy of SADIE&78

Scrambled Eggs with Toast

Ingredients:

- 3-4 eggs equivalent to 1.5 cups when beaten
- 4 tbsp. chunky salsa
- 2 jalapeno peppers
- 2 slices of whole-wheat bread
- Salt and pepper to taste

Directions:

1. Beat up eggs until consistent.
2. Pour beaten eggs into pan.
3. Dice up jalapenos.
4. Add in jalapenos, salsa, and any additional seasoning.
5. Serve on top of toast with salsa on top and enjoy!

Number of servings: 1

Macros:

Total calories: 338.4

Protein: 41.6 g
Carbs: 32.2
Fat: 2.1 g

*Recipe courtesy of SADIE78

High Protein Breakfast Sandwich

Ingredients:

- 1 English muffin
- 1 slice of cheddar cheese
- 1 thin slice of ham
- 1/4 cup of egg whites

Directions:

1. Slice English muffin in half and put in toaster.
2. Microwave egg whites in small bowl for roughly 30 seconds.
3. Stir egg whites in microwave and microwave for additional 5-15 seconds.
4. Layer egg, cheese, and ham in between English muffin halves and enjoy.

Number of servings: 1

Marcos:

Total calories: 217.1

Protein: 22.5 g
Carbs: 25.7 g
Fat: 2.4 g

*Recipe courtesy of CELESTIALAXIS

Banana Vanilla High Protein Soft Serve

Ingredients:

- 1 cup unsweetened coconut milk
- 1 large frozen banana
- 1 scoop vanilla flavored protein powder
- 1 tsp. vanilla extract

Directions:

1. Blend ingredients in blender for 1 ½ minutes.

Number of servings: 1

Macros:

Total calories: 312.2

Protein: 26.3 g
Carbs: 37.6 g
Fat: 6.7 g

*Recipe courtesy of SAPPHIRE983

Protein Lemon Mousse

Ingredients:

- 3 cups fat free cottage cheese
- 1 oz. lemon fat free instant pudding mix
- 1 1/4 cups skim milk

Directions:

1. Put all ingredients and blend until smooth.

Number of servings: 3

Total calories: 171.8

Protein: 30.3 g
Carbs: 12.5 g
Fat: 0.0

*Recipe courtesy of HJSIMM

Chapter 9: Frequently Asked Questions

What if I'm not losing or gaining weight eating 13 calories per pound of bodyweight?

If you've been struggling to lose weight eating 13 calories per pound of bodyweight then I recommend using a different method to set your calories. Before I get into that though, you must first make sure you were actually eating 13 calories per pound of bodyweight minus 500 calories to lose 1 pound per week. It's easy to overestimate the amount of calories you're eating, and this could be the reason why you're not seeing results.

Once you've made sure you've accurately been tracking your calories, you can take your goal bodyweight, multiply it by 11, and then eat that many calories (don't subtract anything from the final calculated number).

Yes, I understand that your goal bodyweight will be a random number that you think you'll look good at, so take your best guess. Start on the higher side and work your way down from there if you still aren't losing weight.

Here's an example for a 250-pound male.

Current Weight 250

Goal Bodyweight 200

200 x 11= 2,200 daily calories

Let's say once this person reaches his goal of 200 pounds, he's still not satisfied with how he looks. From there, he can simply set a new goal bodyweight (i.e. 190 pounds for example) and go from there.

On the other hand, let's say you're struggling to add muscle eating 13 calories per pound of bodyweight plus 250 calories. Again, make sure you're accurately tracking the amount of calories you're eating. You could be miscounting your calories, and that would account for why you're not gaining any weight. Once you've made sure you're tracking things accurately, you can add 100 calories to your total resting metabolic rate weekly until you start gaining weight. For example:

A 180-pound male looking to gain weight would multiply his bodyweight by 13 to determine his maintenance calories.

180 x 13= 2,340

This person would then add 250 calories to 2,340 and get a total of 2,590 calories per day. If he eats 2,590 calories on a daily basis, he should start to gain 0.5 pound per week. However, if he doesn't, he can simply add 100 calories to his original 2,590 calories on a weekly basis until he does.

For example, on week 1, he would eat 2,690 calories. If he didn't gain any weight by the end of the week, he would eat 2,790 calories for the following week, and so on and so forth until he starts gaining weight.

What if I hit a plateau and I stop losing weight at my regular pace?

Let's say you've been losing weight just fine, but then all of the sudden you hit a wall and stop losing weight. In this case, take your new current bodyweight (which should be a lower number from when you first started) and multiply that by 13.

Take that number and subtract 250 from it. This will be your new daily caloric intake for you to lose weight.

This will have you losing weight at a rate of approximately 0.5-pound per week. You may have previously been losing weight at a rate of 1-pound per week, but now you'll lose at a rate of 0.5-pound per week.

This is because I don't want you to drastically reduce your calories all of the sudden, and because if you've hit a plateau, you're likely very close to hitting your goal weight anyway.

How many meals should I eat per day?

You can eat as many meals as you like throughout the day. Meal frequency doesn't matter for weight loss (16), but the total amount of calories you eat does. So eat however is easiest for you and your schedule.

I, myself, prefer to eat 3 meals a day and that works great for most people. However, feel free to eat 6 times per day or even as little as once per day. As long as you're hitting your macros, you'll be fine.

What do I do once I reach my goal bodyweight?

Contrary to what you might be thinking, things aren't going to be that much different from what you've been doing to lose weight. You still need to do flexible dieting and continue eating in the same manner that you previously were. This means that you should still keep the same eating schedule and keep eating similar meals to the ones that you were eating to lose weight.

However, there's one difference between maintenance and creating a caloric deficit to lose weight. The difference is that you get to consume more calories! How many calories? Well, this is pretty easy to figure out as a matter of fact.

Step #1: Determine at what rate you were losing weight (i.e. 1 pound per week)

Step #2: Translate pounds lost per week into calories
    0.5-pound lost per week= 250 calories
    1 pound lost per week= 500 calories
    1.5 pounds lost per week= 750 calories
    2 pounds lost per week= 1,000 calories, etc.

Step #3: Add in those additional calories to what you were previously eating to maintain your new weight.

For example, let's say someone was losing weight at a rate of 1 pound per week by eating 1,850 calories per day. Once he hits his goal weight, he needs to eat 2,350 calories (1,850+500) per day to maintain his new weight.

You'll also need to recalculate your macro percentages. Continuing with this example, this individual would need to do the following with his new caloric intake:

2,350 x .40= 940 daily calories from protein
2,350 x .35= 822.5 daily calories from carbs
2,350 x .25= 587.5 daily calories from fat

How much weight should I lift during the workouts?

Lift as much weight as you possibly can for the given rep range. Initially, you won't know how much weight to use, so you'll have to take your best guess. For example, let's say you're doing bench press for 8 reps. You think you can lift around 150 pounds for that many reps, but on your first set, you easily complete 10 reps.

This means the weight is too light and you need to increase it for the next set. On the next set, you lift 165 pounds and struggle to complete the 8th rep. This is what you want to happen, and it means you've found a good weight to use. Once you can complete all 3 sets for 8 reps with 165 pounds, move up to 170 the next time you bench press. If you can't complete 8 reps for all 3 sets, stick with 165 until you can. Here's an example:

Workout 1: Bench Press with 165 pounds
Set 1: 8 reps
Set 2: 8 reps
Set 3: 7 reps

Because you only completed 7 reps on the last set, stick with 165 for the next workout.

Workout 2: Bench Press with 165 pounds
Set 1: 8 reps
Set 2: 8 reps
Set 3: 8 reps

Because you completed all 3 sets for 8 reps, move up to 170 on your next workout with bench press.

Note: It's better to use a weight that's too heavy and miss a rep or two than it is to use a weight that's too light and leave some reps in the tank. For example, it's better to do 170 pounds and only complete 6 reps instead of 8 as opposed to using 155 pounds and stopping at 8 reps even though you could've easily done more reps.

How Fast Should I Lose Weight?

The more weight you have to lose, the faster the rate at which you can lose the weight. For example, if you have 50+ pounds to lose, you can lose weight at a rate of 2 pounds or more per week. If you only have 5 pounds to lose, then lose weight at a rate of 0.5 pound per week.

For most people, losing 1 pound per week is the sweet spot. You'll be creating an average caloric deficit of 500 calories daily. At this pace, you'll be losing weight fairly quickly, and you won't be miserable all of the time from a complete lack of calories.

How much water should I drink on a daily basis?

Your body is made up of about 60% water so it's important to consume water for several reasons. Drinking water regularly:

- Helps keep your joints and ligaments fluid, which can help prevent injury
- Helps control your caloric intake.
- Flushes out toxins
- Improves skin quality
- Improves kidney function
- Improves your focus

Many people recommend that you should drink 1 gallon of water per day. This is a blanket answer that doesn't meet individual needs. This recommendation would have a 100-pound woman drinking the same amount of water as a 200-pound man. Absurd!

Other health experts advise drinking eight 8-ounce glasses (64 ounces total) of water a day. But again 64 ounces isn't going to be enough for most people. What should you do then? I don't keep track of my water intake—I go by how I feel and the color of my urine.

Your body's own thirst mechanism will be accurate in telling you if you need more water. If you feel thirsty, go drink some water. If not, then you're probably ok. You can also use the color of your urine to judge how hydrated you are. If your urine is yellow, then you should drink more water. If it's clear then you should be good to go. This keeps things simple and it's one less thing you have to keep track of.

Are there any supplements that you recommend I take?

Most supplements are a complete waste of money. There's not a single supplement that's required in order for you to build muscle or burn fat. In fact, I advise for the first 6 weeks of your IIFYM diet that you don't take *any* supplements at all.

This is because I want you to see for yourself that it really is possible for you to get results without supplements. Your hard work and dedication matter way more than any pill or powder.

With that being said, there are a few supplements I recommend if you have the budget for them:

#1: Protein Powder:

You can't have a recommended list of supplements without protein powder on the list right? Just kidding. But this has to be one of the most overhyped supplements of all time.

I think that the media does a really good job of making us believe that we must take protein powder to build muscle or take it to prevent muscle loss. I do think that protein powder can provide some benefits if *you need it.*

If you struggle to consistently hit your macros with protein then I would consider investing in a protein powder. Protein is necessary to help build and prevent the breakdown of muscle.

Therefore, ensuring that your muscle is spared is a good thing. However, don't go out of your way and eat more calories just for the sake of consuming more protein.

#2: Fish/Krill Oil

These oils are great sources of Omega-3 fatty acids. This is a good thing because most people consume too many Omega-6 fatty acids with foods like vegetable and canola oil.

Ideally, you want to be consuming a 1 to 1 ratio of Omega-3's to Omega-6's. Fish and krill oil can help you narrow the gap between the two types of fatty acids that you're consuming.

The main benefit from consuming these oils is that they act as an anti-inflammatory in your body. When you consume Omega-6's on the other hand, they act as an inflammatory.

That's why it's important to strike a balance with both of the fatty acids. The anti-inflammatory benefit is great because it can reduce your risk of developing heart disease or high blood pressure.

Finally, reducing inflammation can aid in muscle recovery. If you're going to invest in fish or krill oil, make sure that it's a very high-grade supplement.

The way that some of the lower quality oils are processed inhibits the absorption of them, which would make them completely useless. As for investing in fish or krill oil, taking either one is fine really.

Krill oil does contain the antioxidant astaxanthin (17), which helps with joint health, boosts cognitive function and helps promote a healthy cholesterol balance, while fish oil does not. However, I have noticed that krill oil can be harder to find, and it's typically more expensive so don't sweat not buying it.

#3: Digestive Enzymes

This is my favorite supplement of all time, and it's probably one of the most underrated supplements as well. If your body can't absorb the vitamins and nutrients that you're consuming then what's the point?

The sad fact of the matter is that when our foods get cooked, many of the enzymes get destroyed. Digestive enzymes will not only help to replenish those enzymes missed from cooked foods, but it will also help your body to better break down and utilize the nutrients that you're eating.

Also, if you ever suffer regularly from bloating, heartburn, or have bad skin, give digestive enzymes a try and see if you notice a difference. Of course, it's important to note that these enzymes need to be high quality if you want them to be of any use.

Simply going to the local grocery store and purchasing a $10 bottle of enzymes isn't going to cut it. You must buy a high-quality enzyme if you want to get any use out of it. Personally, I recommend using Bio Trust.

How Do I Motivate Myself to Go to the Gym?

Finding the motivation to go to the gym or eat right can be hard. No matter who you are, there will be times when you don't feel like working out. Having that feeling is ok, but you can't let it control you. There will be times when you'll have to do it anyway even when you don't feel like it.

That's what will ultimately separate a long-term successful fitness journey from failing at it. I do have some tips to help you out along the way however:

Tip #1: Focus on Gradual Improvements

Many people make fitness an all-or-nothing game. They tell themselves that they'll workout 5 days a week and eat clean 100% of the time for the rest of their lives. Let's say you workout only 4 days one week. Are you a failure?

Of course not. You still worked out 4 days, but in your mind you are because you failed to reach 5 workouts. You make it hard to celebrate any small successes that you do have because the standards are too high.

Instead, focus on making smaller, more gradual improvements, and celebrate any successes you have along the way. For example, start off with a goal to only workout 2 days per week if it's been years since you've last worked out. Once you achieve that goal, you'll feel good about yourself, and you can move up to working out 3 days per week and so on.

Tip #2: Action Leads Motivation

People think they have to get the inspiration or motivation from somewhere in order to take the action necessary to workout. The reverse of that is actually true. You need to start by taking an action no matter how small. And once you get started, you'll likely want to continue on with what you're doing.

When I think about everything I have to do to workout such as put my gym clothes on, drive to the gym, workout with a bunch of grueling exercises, drive back and shower, I start to make up silly excuses as to why I should skip this time. Instead, I'll tell myself to do just one exercise when I get to the gym and not pressure myself to do anything more. After I finish that first exercise, it's always easier for me to finish the rest of the workout.

You just have to get started. Try this out for any healthy habit you want to start. For example, if you want to start flossing your teeth, tell yourself you'll only floss one tooth and don't pressure yourself to do anything more than that!

Tip #3: Put Your Own Money on the Line

Money is a very powerful motivator. And you can use your own money to motivate yourself to start working out more. Here's what you're going to do—give someone a good amount of money. Not $20, but something that would actually hurt you—$100, $200, $500, or whatever you can't afford to lose.

Then tell your friend that if you don't go to the gym 3 days this week, for example, they get to keep the money. When you give up the money in the first place, you'll fight to get it back. This is much different than telling yourself you'll give the money to someone after you miss your workouts.

It's too easy to make an excuse and not give away the money. Give the money up in the first place and make sure your friend actually holds you accountable to it. This is by far the best way to get motivation to workout. There's a real cost involved if you don't comply. You'll either get ripped or go broke trying.

Conclusion:

Thanks for getting this book and reading it all the way through to the end! If It Fits Your Macros is an easy way to get and stay in shape for the rest of your life. You simply have to stay dedicated. Flexible dieting will work as long as you put forth the needed effort.

Feel free to email me any questions you may have about fitness at thomas@rohmerfitness.com

And finally, if this book was helpful, please take a few minutes and leave a review. Your feedback will help me make better content for you in the future!

Sources

(1) Stote KS, Baer DJ, Spears K, Paul DR, Harris GK, et al. A controlled trial of reduced meal frequency without caloric restriction in healthy, normal-weight, middle aged men. AM J Clin Nutr 2007;85:981-988.

(2) Louis M, Poortmans JR, Francaux M, Hultman E, Berre J, et al. Creatine supplementation has no effect on human muscle protein turnover at rest in the postabsorptive or fed states. Am J Physiol Endocrinol Metab:284;765-770. Nutritional Supplements in the U.S. Packaged Facts. November 1, 2006

(3) Cureton KJ, Collins MA, Hill DW, et al. Muscle hypertrophy in men and women. Med Sci Sport Exerc 1988; 20:338-44.

(4) https://www.ncbi.nlm.nih.gov/pubmed/19345947

(5) https://www.ncbi.nlm.nih.gov/pubmed/22825659

(6)
https://www.ncbi.nlm.nih.gov/pubmed/11255140

(7)
https://www.ncbi.nlm.nih.gov/pubmed/19927027

(8)
https://www.ncbi.nlm.nih.gov/books/NBK21190/

(9)
http://www.cnn.com/2010/HEALTH/11/08/twinkie.diet.professor/

(10)
https://www.ncbi.nlm.nih.gov/pmc/articles/PMC4836564/

(11)
http://www.internettime.com/2015/08/writing-down-your-learning-goals-increases-the-odds-you-will-accomplish-them-by-42/

(12) http://elitedaily.com/money/writing-down-your-goals/1068863/

(13)
http://www.dominican.edu/dominicannews/study-highlights-strategies-for-achieving-goals

(14) http://lifehacker.com/5738093/why-you-learn-more-effectively-by-writing-than-typing

(15) http://www.influenceatwork.com/wp-content/uploads/2012/02/E_Brand_principles.pdf

(16) https://www.ncbi.nlm.nih.gov/pubmed/26024494

(17) https://en.wikipedia.org/wiki/Astaxanthin

*Recipes courtesy of users at sparkpeople.com

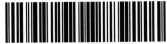

Made in the USA
San Bernardino, CA
29 August 2017